Homemade Healing Salve:
10 Tutorials on How to Make a Herbal Salve And Top 15 Recipes

Table of content

Introduction

The fact that you're reading this book shows that you have an interest in natural medicine, or at least hate to use chemicals or other standard medicine, which can often be smelly and for some, equally scary.

If you've done any research into herbal remedies and natural medicine, you've likely encountered quackery and pseudo-scientific based recipes for every ailment under the sun.

The simple fact is that you cannot cure everything with an herbal salve, or even most ailments. More importantly, it's no substitute for a real doctor and diagnoses, so if you're not sure what your health concern is, please see a real doctor and get proper treatment.

That said, herbs, *do* possesses real medicinal properties. The trick is to find out what those properties are and how to do use those benefits safely. This book will guide you on the path and provide you with real recipes that you can use for specific ailments backed by science.

You'll learn what works, what doesn't, how best to make your salves, and what are the best and most reliable uses for herbal salves. More importantly, you'll learn some really simple and cool ways to spice us (pun intended) your herbal salve shelf at home.

You have probably seen many site selling salves claiming they can cure everything from cancer or chronic pain. If that's the reason you want to make the salve, go see a doctor instead.

The recipes provided here will be broken down into two primary categories. The first is for alleviating skin dryness (which can support healing for things like psoriasis and seborrheic dermatitis) and added moisturizing. The second is for cuts, burns, scrapes, and insect bites. A good smelling salve is an added benefit for both of the aforementioned groups.

Chapter 1 – Tips For Beginners (and Those who Aren't Sure)

Tip #1 Seek a Medical Professional When in Doubt.

If you've had a lingering serious or chronic medical issues that hasn't healed and everything you've tried has had minimal help, please see a doctor first for a proper diagnosis. That also goes for a new illness that you just discovered. If your issue is something other than a minor ailment, don't try to treat yourself or guess at your diagnosis or the best treatment; see a professional right away.

I realize that you may want to do everything on your own the natural way, but remember that just because something isn't natural, doesn't make it safe, and there is no substitute for a licensed medical doctor. Diagnose the problem first, and then listen to your doctor's advice for what is and isn't safe. After that, feel free to experiment with what works best for your particular issue. If someone tries to convince you otherwise, ignore them, and walk away.

Tip #2 Know What You're Getting Before Your Buy it.

Several studies were conducted that looked at the ingredients of salves or other natural medical and herbal remedies with startling results showed that most natural medicines and supplements did not contain the ingredients that they claimed to contain. Keep in mind that the ingredients *are* drugs, whether they are natural or not. As a result, when you purchase "natural" items that are already prepackaged, they often contain fillers instead of the ingredients that are supposed to contain.

What this means is that you don't want to purchase any prepackaged natural items. The rate of false ingredients is so high, above 80%, they you cannot reliable purchase any prepackaged item as a means of a short cut to your salve.

If you want to make your own herbal salve, you'll need to do it from scratch buy starting with all the ingredients, one by one, instead of purchased salves that are prepackaged or using ingredients that are already processed or partially processed. In other words, buy each ingredient separately.

Tip #3 Know Who You're Buying From Before Your Buy it.

With tip #2 in mind, you'll also want to insure that your individual ingredients are what they say they are. This means you need to do two things. The first is that you need to know the reputation of the retailer or person from who you are making the purchase. It also means that you need to investigate the reputation of the person or company that is selling you the individual product.

I know this process can feel like it's taking all the fun out of a do it yourself project, but it will be even less fun, if after all your hard work and excitement, you find that you've been duped. Don't leave your herbal salve to chance. Look up customer reviews to see what other people have said about the seller, and remember the old adage: If looks too good to be true, it probably is.

What this means for you, is that if you know an essential oil costs $10 for a milliliter, and you find an outfit selling it for 50 cents a milliliter, something is usually amiss. Don't let greed or the desire to save a few bucks trick you into getting swindled and wasting all or your money, or worse, getting injured from a dangerous ingredient that may cause reactions. Be smart, and always play it safe.

Tip #4 Purchase Your Ingredients in Known Concentrations.

Unless you are an expert at extraction and can create things like essential oils accurately and consistently, it's always best to purchase the essential oil or raw ingredients in their concentrated form. The reason is that if you want to make an herbal salve, the concentrations vary dramatically when you are using the raw plants and un-extracted materials.

In practical terms, this means that your herbal salve may not only be ineffective, but it could also be dangerous if you have dramatically higher concentrations than you expect. If you want your topical solution to be 2% of your active ingredient and it ends up being 10%, that can mean the difference between having a soothing and beneficial intended effect to having one of great irritation, and in some cases danger.

I won't go into all the scientific reasons why the above issue is the case, but if you understand it, it will make your recipes for herbal salves more effective and safer, and that's what you want.

If you do decide to extract the active ingredients are your own, make sure you have the process down before you use any of your ingredients. Make sure that you create a specific system, and that you use the system to insure that your ingredients will also be as close to the same as possible each time you make them.

Tip #5 Practice Makes Perfect.

Don't expect your perfect batch to be perfection. If you go in knowing that you will likely screw things up, you'll make things easier on yourself. That being the case, know you will likely create an inferior salve the first few tries, don't use all your ingredients at once. Don't create one enormous batch, only to have to scrap it until you get it correct.

Start with the smallest amount possible to test out both the process and the effectiveness of your salve. Also, start with the cheapest salve for your intended purpose. If you have a few recipes, start with the cheaper one first, so that you get a handle on the process and system of what you are doing. If you combine the use of a small scale sample to test your sample and the use of a cheap recipe, you'll save yourself a lot of money, and you will likely stay more motivated to push through until you come up with a product that you like and works best for you.

Tip #6 Research the effectiveness of your active ingredient.

The recipes provided in this book have done the hard work and research for you for those specific recipes and ailments, but if you want to try something different on your own, do more than just a simple Google search to see if your particular active ingredient works for your particular use.

The best way to research is by searching for what *doesn't* work. When you look for scientific based research that uses a skeptical eye on natural medicine, you will get a much more accurate picture of what your salves can actually do and what they can't do. Natural medicine, and those that sell it are in the business of selling it. You will be promised a cure for everything under the sun, but look at the evidence, not the empty promises, before you set out to make your salve. When in doubt, go back to tip #1.

Tip #7 Make a Plan.

I usually put making a plan as the first thing to do before you get started, but in this case, please review tips one through six first. Before you can make a proper plan, you want to make sure that you have to tools and knowledge in place to attack your recipes and your goals safely and with the right ingredients.

The key to any plan is to first identify the why. What is the reason why you want to make your herbal salve? Is it for a specific skin ailment? Is it for moisturizing? Do you want to smell better or to alleviate psoriasis or both? If you've followed steps one through five, you probably already know the why, but if you don't, put that down first before you start the rest of the plan.

Once you have down the why, list all your recipes, ingredients as well as the concentrations, supplier, and instructions on how to make your salve. I would also recommend that you have at least two trusted suppliers for each ingredient, just in case one is out of stock.

The next step to making a plan is to have a list of trusted resources for when you begin your preparation. This is especially crucial when you're first starting out and you need to work out any kinks before you really get going.

Tip #8 Replace the Base

The base of any herbal salve is usually some type of oil, many times, you'll see that extra virgin olive oil is a key ingredient. While the olive oil may hold your salve together and serve as an adequate moisturizer, there are better choices. You'll notice a variety of bases that I use in my recipes, but feel free to experiment with what smells and feels right for you.

The base is not the active ingredient, so it usually won't change the effectiveness of your herbal salve if you switch out olive oil, for say coconut or agave nectar, or some other better smelling substance that can do the trick.

Tip #9 Watch Someone Else do it First.

If you haven't done this before, or the particular recipe your trying out, look up some informational or instructional videos of a trusted source who has done it. If you can watch a person do it live, great. If not, an instructional video will still be a tremendous help before you get started on actually putting the ingredients together.

You should also watch more than one person or more than one video. It's good to get a different perspective, and you'll often learn additional things that one person may miss in their instruction. Some videos may show you the incorrect way, or may be amateurish, so watch a few short videos so you can get a variety of perspectives before you begin your endeavor.

Tip #10 Test Your Salve.

Hopefully, you've followed the other tips, you've researched, started out small, and started with the cheapest salve. At this point, you want to test it, just like you would any harsh chemical on a carpet, or any topical medication. Each person has their own set of genes and reactions to medications, including natural medication such as essential oils. As such, use a small amount and apply topically before you apply a larger amount.

Using a small amount will allow to see if there is any reaction or undesirable irritation. If there is, don't apply any more. If there is a severe reaction, I recommend seeing a doctor immediately just in case there is some other underlying issue as well as to note the potential allergen so you can avoid it in the future.

Bonus Tip #1 Test Your Equipment and Storage Containers.

Make things easy on yourself by testing your equipment ahead of time before you get started. Don't let a non-working burner, or a cracked container stop you midway through the process, forcing you to waste all of your money and hard work. Checks your supplies ahead of time, and make sure you are good to go.

You should also check your ingredients. If you think something is off about your ingredients, trust your gut. If they look or smell is off, don't you them. Even you purchased from a trusted source, something things fall through the cracks or a good supplier goes bad. When in doubt, throw it out.

Bonus Tip #2 Clean up and Store Your Salve Properly.

Cleaning is essential both before and after your process of making your herbal salve. If your containers are tainted, your salve will be tainted as well. If your cooking instruments contain residue from other recipes, that residue will alter the results and impact of your new salve. Always clean thoroughly before and after your process. If you don't, you risk contamination and danger, making it difficult to determine the cause if you have a reaction in the testing phase of your herbal salve.

Bonus Tip #3 Always Tell Your Doctor About Any Natural Medicine You Use.

Herbal salves, as well as any other natural medicine, contains drugs. When you see your doctor, always tell them what you've applied to your skin and body, even if it's natural and you made it yourself. Essential oils and other ingredients can have reactions to synthetic or normally prescribed medications, so tell your doctor everything about your herbal salves regardless of how minor you think your salve or your condition is.

Bonus Tip #4 Grind Your Herbs.

If you decide to go the do it yourself route on extraction, you'll need to make sure that your herbs are as finely ground as possible. If there are pockets of air, the concentrations will vary significantly. Different techniques can allow you to reduce those air pockets and increase the surface area. I always recommend grinding your herbs at least three times, and then using a filter process to sort out the larger granules of herbs.

Chapter 3 – Herbal Salves For Dry and Damaged Skin.

The healing property of any moisturizer works by adding lipids (fats) to your skin. You can apply just about any type of fat or oil, and it will have some measurable improvement. The key is that all oils are not created equally. Some are better than others. The effectiveness your salve that you use to treat your skin condition or moisturize your skin will vary based on your genetic profile as well as the other ingredients in your salve. I recommend you try all of them, and try different variations of oils based on what works and what is pleasant for you. For skin, rehhmannia, glycyrrhiza glabra, and pontentilla chinensis have been shown to have the best impact on improves skin irritation.

Recipe #1. Coconut Base.

Use five parts of coconut oil to one of beeswax. For your herbal mix, use one part rehmannia.

Use low heat to melt both together. They should be completely blended. Simply stir slowly until there are no visible differences you can see. The next step is to add your herbs. If you read my bonus tip #4, you'll see that you will need to make sure that your herbs are fully ground and extracted if you chose to extract them yourself. Stir the mixture together thoroughly and let cool.

Recipe #2. Coconut Base.

Use four parts of coconut oil to two of beeswax. For your herbal mix, use one part rehmannia.

Use low heat to melt both together. They should be completely blended. Simply stir slowly until there are no visible differences you can see. The next step is to add your herbs. If you read my bonus tip #4, you'll see that you will need to make sure that your herbs are fully ground and extracted if you chose to extract them yourself. Stir the mixture together thoroughly and let cool.

Recipe #3. Coconut Base.

Use three parts of lanolin, two parts coconut oil to one of beeswax. For your herbal mix, use one part rehmannia.

Use low heat to melt both together. They should be completely blended. Simply stir slowly until there are no visible differences you can see. The next step is to add your herbs. If you read my bonus tip #4, you'll see that you will need to make sure that your herbs are fully ground and extracted if you chose to extract them yourself. Stir the mixture together thoroughly and let cool.

Recipe #4. Coconut Base.

Use four parts of lanolin, one-part coconut oil, and two of beeswax. For your herbal mix, use one part rehmannia.

Use low heat to melt both together. They should be completely blended. Simply stir slowly until there are no visible differences you can see. The next step is to add your herbs. If you read my bonus tip #4, you'll see that you will need to make sure that your herbs are fully ground and extracted if you chose to extract them yourself. Stir the mixture together thoroughly and let cool.

Recipe #5. Coconut Base.

Use five parts of coconut oil to one of beeswax. For your herbal mix, use one part glycyrrhiza glabra.

Use low heat to melt both together. They should be completely blended. Simply stir slowly until there are no visible differences you can see. The next step is to add your herbs. If you read my bonus tip #4, you'll see that you will need to make sure that your herbs are fully ground and extracted if you chose to extract them yourself. Stir the mixture together thoroughly and let cool.

Recipe #6. Coconut Base.

Use four parts of coconut oil to two of beeswax. For your herbal mix, use one part glycyrrhiza glabra.

Use low heat to melt both together. They should be completely blended. Simply stir slowly until there are no visible differences you can see. The next step is to add your herbs. If you read my bonus tip #4, you'll see that you will need to make sure that your herbs are fully ground and extracted if you chose to extract them yourself. Stir the mixture together thoroughly and let cool.

Recipe #7. Coconut Base.

Use three parts of lanolin, two parts coconut oil to one of beeswax. For your herbal mix, use one part glycyrrhiza glabra.

Use low heat to melt both together. They should be completely blended. Simply stir slowly until there are no visible differences you can see. The next step is to add your herbs. If you read my bonus tip #4, you'll see that you will need to make sure that your herbs are fully ground and extracted if you chose to extract them yourself. Stir the mixture together thoroughly and let cool.

Recipe #8. Coconut Base.

Use four parts of lanolin, one-part coconut oil, and two of beeswax. For your herbal mix, use one part glycyrrhiza glabra.

Use low heat to melt both together. They should be completely blended. Simply stir slowly until there are no visible differences you can see. The next step is to add your herbs. If you read my bonus tip #4, you'll see that you will need to make sure that your herbs are fully ground and extracted if you chose to extract them yourself. Stir the mixture together thoroughly and let cool.

Chapter 4 – Skin irritation from cuts, bites, and burns.

With skin irritation from cuts, bites, and burns, Aloe-Vera is one of the best proven natural antiseptics out there. Honey is also another ancient antiseptic. Use both more maximum effect.

Recipe #9. Aloe-Vera Base.

Use five parts of Aloe-Vera to one of beeswax. For your herbal mix, use one part pontentilla chinensis.

Use low heat to melt both together. They should be completely blended. Simply stir slowly until there are no visible differences you can see. The next step is to add your herbs. If you read my bonus tip #4, you'll see that you will need to make sure that your herbs are fully ground and extracted if you chose to extract them yourself. Stir the mixture together thoroughly and let cool.

Recipe #10. Aloe-Vera.

Use four parts of Aloe-Vera to two of beeswax. For your herbal mix, use one part rehmannia.

Use low heat to melt both together. They should be completely blended. Simply stir slowly until there are no visible differences you can see. The next step is to add your herbs. If you read my bonus tip #4, you'll see that you will need to make sure that your herbs are fully ground and extracted if you chose to extract them yourself. Stir the mixture together thoroughly and let cool.

Recipe #11. Aloe-Vera.

Use three parts of lanolin, two parts Aloe-Vera to one of beeswax. For your herbal mix, use one part rehmannia.

Use low heat to melt both together. They should be completely blended. Simply stir slowly until there are no visible differences you can see. The next step is to add your herbs. If you read my bonus tip #4, you'll see that you will need to make sure that your herbs are fully ground and extracted if you chose to extract them yourself. Stir the mixture together thoroughly and let cool.

Recipe #12. Aloe-Vera.

Use four parts of lanolin, one-part Aloe-Vera, and two of beeswax. For your herbal mix, use one part pontentilla chinensis.

Use low heat to melt both together. They should be completely blended. Simply stir slowly until there are no visible differences you can see. The next step is to add your herbs. If you read my bonus tip #4, you'll see that you will need to make sure that your herbs are fully ground and extracted if you chose to extract them yourself. Stir the mixture together thoroughly and let cool.

Recipe #13. Aloe-Vera Base.

Use five parts of Aloe-Vera to one of beeswax. For your herbal mix, use one part glycyrrhiza glabra.

Use low heat to melt both together. They should be completely blended. Simply stir slowly until there are no visible differences you can see. The next step is to add your herbs. If you read my bonus tip #4, you'll see that you will need to make sure that your herbs are fully ground and extracted if you chose to extract them yourself. Stir the mixture together thoroughly and let cool.

Recipe #14. Aloe-Vera Base.

Use four parts of Aloe-Vera to two of beeswax. For your herbal mix, use one part glycyrrhiza glabra.

Use low heat to melt both together. They should be completely blended. Simply stir slowly until there are no visible differences you can see. The next step is to add your herbs. If you read my bonus tip #4, you'll see that you will need to make sure that your herbs are fully ground and extracted if you chose to extract them yourself. Stir the mixture together thoroughly and let cool.

Recipe #15. Aloe-Vera Base.

Use three parts of lanolin, two parts Aloe-Vera to one of beeswax. For your herbal mix, use one part glycyrrhiza glabra.

Use low heat to melt both together. They should be completely blended. Simply stir slowly until there are no visible differences you can see. The next step is to add your herbs. If you read my bonus tip #4, you'll see that you will need to make sure that your herbs are fully ground and extracted if you chose to extract them yourself. Stir the mixture together thoroughly and let cool.

Bonus Recipe #1 Aloe-Vera Base.

Use four parts of lanolin, one-part Aloe-Vera, and two of beeswax. For your herbal mix, use one part pontentilla chinensis.

Use low heat to melt both together. They should be completely blended. Simply stir slowly until there are no visible differences you can see. The next step is to add your herbs. If you read my bonus tip #4, you'll see that you will need to make sure that your herbs are fully ground and extracted if you chose to extract them yourself. Stir the mixture together thoroughly and let cool.

Bonus Recipe #2 Aloe-Vera Base.

Use four parts of lanolin, one-part Aloe-Vera, and two of beeswax. For your herbal mix, use one part pontentilla chinensis.

Use low heat to melt both together. They should be completely blended. Simply stir slowly until there are no visible differences you can see. The next step is to add your herbs. If you read my bonus tip #4, you'll see that you will need to make sure that your herbs are fully ground and extracted if you chose to extract them yourself. Stir the mixture together thoroughly and let cool.

Finally, after you let your mixture cool, and one-part honey. Make sure that your honey is the unpasteurized version so it retains its full properties.

Bonus Recipe #3 Aloe-Vera Base.

Use three parts of lanolin, two-part Aloe-Vera, and two of beeswax. For your herbal mix, use one part glycyrrhiza glabra.

Use low heat to melt both together. They should be completely blended. Simply stir slowly until there are no visible differences you can see. The next step is to add your herbs. If you read my bonus tip #4, you'll see that you will need to make sure that your herbs are fully ground and extracted if you chose to extract them yourself. Stir the mixture together thoroughly and let cool.

Finally, after you let your mixture cool, and one-part honey. Make sure that your honey is the unpasteurized version so it retains its full properties.

Bonus Recipe #4 Aloe-Vera Base.

Use one parts of lanolin, four-part Aloe-Vera, and two of beeswax. For your herbal mix, use one part glycyrrhiza glabra.

Use low heat to melt both together. They should be completely blended. Simply stir slowly until there are no visible differences you can see. The next step is to add your herbs. If you read my bonus tip #4, you'll see that you will need to make sure that your herbs are fully ground and extracted if you chose to extract them yourself. Stir the mixture together thoroughly and let cool.

Finally, after you let your mixture cool, and one-part honey. Make sure that your honey is the unpasteurized version so it retains its full properties.

Bonus Recipe #5 Aloe-Vera Base.

Use two parts of lanolin, two-part Aloe-Vera, and three of beeswax. For your herbal mix, use one part pontentilla chinensis.

Use low heat to melt both together. They should be completely blended. Simply stir slowly until there are no visible differences you can see. The next step is to add your herbs. If you read my bonus tip #4, you'll see that you will need to make sure that your herbs are fully ground and extracted if you chose to extract them yourself. Stir the mixture together thoroughly and let cool.

Finally, after you let your mixture cool, and one-part honey. Make sure that your honey is the unpasteurized version so it retains its full properties.

Bonus Recipe #6 Aloe-Vera Base.

Use two parts of lanolin, two-part Aloe-Vera, and four of beeswax. For your herbal mix, use one part pontentilla chinensis.

Use low heat to melt both together. They should be completely blended. Simply stir slowly until there are no visible differences you can see. The next step is to add your herbs. If you read my bonus tip #4, you'll see that you will need to make sure that your herbs are fully ground and extracted if you chose to extract them yourself. Stir the mixture together thoroughly and let cool.

Finally, after you let your mixture cool, and one-part honey. Make sure that your honey is the unpasteurized version so it retains its full properties.

Bonus Recipe #7 Aloe-Vera Base.

Use two parts of lanolin, two-part Aloe-Vera, and four of beeswax. For your herbal mix, use ½ part rehhmannia, ½ part glycyrrhiza glabra, and ½ part pontentilla.

Use low heat to melt both together. They should be completely blended. Simply stir slowly until there are no visible differences you can see. The next step is to add your herbs. If you read my bonus tip #4, you'll see that you will need to make sure that your herbs are fully ground and extracted if you chose to extract them yourself. Stir the mixture together thoroughly and let cool.

Finally, after you let your mixture cool, and one-part honey. Make sure that your honey is the unpasteurized version so it retains its full properties.

Conclusion

I hope you've enjoyed reading about the different recipes. Don't forget that you can almost always switch out the base for other desired ingredients. The main thing is that you first identify why you are using the salve, and research the effectiveness of the salve before you begin.

Seek medical attention if you have a serious issue, and always use a trusted source for your supplies and active ingredients. Follow the same process and system whenever you begin, which means that you must first plan before you start. As long as you follow those steps, you'll enjoy the fun and easy process of making you wonderful and hopefully great smelling herbal salves.